I0408157

Oregano Essential Oil

Benefits, Properties, Applications, Studies & Recipes

by Ann Sullivan

Published in USA by:

Ann Sullivan
217 N. Seacrest Blvd #9
Boynton Beach
FL 33425

© Copyright 2015

ISBN-13: 978-1545428351
ISBN-10: 1545428352

ALL RIGHTS RESERVED. No part of this publication may be reproduced or transmitted in any form whatsoever, electronic, or mechanical, including photocopying, recording, or by any informational storage or retrieval system without express written, dated and signed permission from the author.

TABLE OF CONTENTS

Introduction

What are essential oils, and how might they be used for therapeutic purposes?

Essential oils are ultra-potent oils, extracted from plants and flowers that have been utilized in medicine for centuries. Presently, they're most commonly used to supplement pharmaceutical medication, but they can also be an effective alternative to pharmaceuticals in the event that you don't have access to them. Before you dismiss essential oils as a means to support the body's natural defenses against injuries and illness, take a look at the historical evidence of the oils' medicinal competence in practice. Your average age-old medical text will demonstrate that essential oils, herbs, and plenty of other natural ingredients have, for thousands of years, successfully enhanced immune function to meet and defeat any number of ailments and injuries. Though traditional medicine is considered "alternative" now, it was once the gold standard. And, frankly, perhaps it still should be, as these natural age-tested remedies can fortify the body's battlements against everything from simple maladies, like headaches, cuts and bruises, to serious diseases, like cancer.

Essential oils are deemed "essential," because the oils are composed of the "essence" of the plant. The difference between essential oils and other oils – like olive oil or vegetable oil, for instance – is that essential oils have high volatility and reduced fixation, which results in faster evaporation, enabling their popular use in aromatherapy. Even at high temperatures, olive and vegetable oils don't evaporate.

Essential oils are especially necessary when it comes to a major natural or man-made disaster or some potential viral outbreak. In these types of dire situations, you may not have quick access (or any access at all) to your standard pharmaceutical supply; so essential oils, along with other alternative medicines, will be your go-to health aids in the case of social collapse, viral outbreak or devastating natural disaster. When medical access is null and void, alternatives to our modern-day standard are the only chance we have to keep pathogens at bay.

You probably don't realize that you already use essential oils every day. They're in perfumes, shampoos, soaps, ointments...they're even used in furniture polish. Why are they found in so many aromatic products? Well, basically, because essential oils are super concentrated aromatic liquids, so their scent is remarkably strong. Let's put this into perspective: to steam tea, you use a few leaves of peppermint or juniper; to produce a single ounce of essential oil, five whole *pounds* of peppermint or juniper leaves are required. Some sources claim that to produce twelve pounds of essential oil would necessitate an acre of peppermint, juniper, or any other oil you're looking to produce en masse. Unlike vegetable oil, you don't often find concentrated therapeutic-grade essential oils sold by the tubload; instead the oils are often sold in easily carried small, dark bottles, perfect for your GOOD bag (Get Out Of Dodge). Which is exactly what this book is aiming to help you do – get out of dodge with your most vital of essential oils intact, in particular a good supply of oregano essential oil.

Why oregano, you ask? Well, in order to get you quickly up to speed on this most essential of oils, below we've provided a condensed synopsis of oregano, after which we'll outline in greater detail the oil's history, properties, and common therapeutic uses, so that you – the consumer – might have a better understanding of the oil's benefits and applications. We've even provided supportive remedies for pure oregano, as well as blended recipes that incorporate the valuable oil. Chapter 3 will further detail past scientific research on oregano essential oil.

Now, let's get down to it – **Essential Oil 101: the Basics of Oregano.**

Summary: Oregano, or Origanum compactum, has traditionally been used for cooking. Of course, its medicinal properties push this oil beyond the mere seasoning of the odd dish. Oregano has incredible antioxidant, immune-boosting, and respiratory supportive properties.

When choosing your oregano essential oil, it is important to know that there are a number of variations of the oregano species and several specific chemotypes, many of which are not medicinal. As these different species have grown in different climates, the chemical properties of each chemotype have been altered. Having different properties means that differing chemotypes of oregano can be used for different health issues. Keep in mind that the CT Carvacrol chemotype is the one you should be after for therapeutic purposes.

Description: Oregano oil is commonly extracted through steam distillation. The leaves, flowers and buds are most often used. The oil is pale yellow in color, thin in consistency, and has a strong sharp, herbaceous scent.

Uses: Beyond those applications previously mentioned, additional uses for oregano essential oil include supporting the body's natural defenses against colds, flu, coughs, digestion, diarrhea, yeast infection and sore throat. It can also be used as a disinfectant and immune booster. When it comes to mood and emotion, oregano can provide a sense of safety and security.

Properties: Antibiotic, antiviral, antibacterial, antifungal, anti-inflammatory, anti-allergenic, antiparasitic, digestive, emmenagogue, expectorant, and disinfectant.

Application: Dilute 1:3 with a carrier oil. You can apply topically, diffuse or use as a dietary supplement.

Safety Precautions: Oregano has been approved by the FDA for internal consumption and so can be used as a dietary supplement. However, if pregnant, breastfeeding or diabetic, consult a physician before using this oil. If you have sensitive skin, dilute heavily or avoid. Be cautious if inhaling directly.

Fun facts: Oregano is derived from the Greek phrase "joy of the mountain," which is "oreganos." The Greeks used this oil to remedy hemlock poisoning and venomous bites.

Oregano is also one of the herbs found in the first herbalist's record of remedies. Hildegrad of Bingen lived from 1098 to 1179, and during her lifetime, she compiled over 12,000 remedies into her self-titled Medicine Book.

Chapter 1:
Benefits of Oregano Essential Oil

We wouldn't be recommending the use of oregano essential oil if it wasn't beneficial, but you may be wondering what, exactly, these benefits are. In this chapter, we'll take a closer look at oregano and its many uses.

What is Oregano?

Oregano is a plant, the leaf of which has long been used for culinary purposes, as well as medicinal applications. Oregano has primarily been used to combat gastrointestinal issues, respiratory tract issues, and viral issues.

Due to its love of hot and somewhat dry climates, the genus of the mint family, Origanum vulgare, is native to the Mediterranean region and southwest Europe, and is the most common species of oregano. The perennial herb produces purple flowers and is sometimes called 'sweet marjoram' and, indeed, is related to the herb, marjoram.

Historically, oregano has been utilized by everyone from traditional Austrian shamen to famous Greek physicians. Hippocrates, known as the "father of western medicine," used oregano to protect against respiratory and gastrointestinal issues, as well as in application as an antiseptic. Often taken in tea or as an ointment, traditional Austrian medicine applied oregano for both internal and external uses to support the body's natural defenses against respiratory, gastrointestinal, and nervous issues.

In Food

If you've ever eaten pizza, then it's likely you've partaken in this culinary herb. Oregano leaves flavor its foods with an aromatic, somewhat bitter taste. For culinary purposes, the herb is better dried than fresh and is considered higher quality if its strength nearly numbs the tongue. Oregano's quality varies according to seasonal changes, as well as the climate and soil in which it's cultivated. The herb, as can be expected, is popularly used in other Italian dishes as well, including pasta and roasted or grilled vegetables, fish and meat; although, oregano is more commonly used in southern Italy, while marjoram is preferred in the north.

But when it comes to culinary spices, the Italians certainly don't hold a monopoly over oregano; Latin American, Spanish, Greek, Egyptian, Turkish, Philippine, and Palestinian cuisines (and many more) all use this spice generously. The Greeks use it in their salad, accompanied by lemon and olive oil. The Turkish use it to flavor meat, especially when seasoning kebabs. And the Philippines use oregano to yield flavor to boiled water buffalo, while simultaneously combating the odor.

Subspecies

Man has developed a number of different oregano strains and subspecies over the years, each of which offer unique properties and flavors, from spicy to sweet. We've identified some of the most popular subspecies below.

Origanum vulgare, subspecies gracile, is characterized by glossy leaves and pink flowers, which is why it is more often used for ornamental purposes than other subspecies of oregano. Grown in Pakistan, Iran, Afghanistan, Turkey and Central Asia, this subspecies offers a spicy, pungent flavor.

Origanum vulgare, subspecies glandulosum, has been shown to have DPPH radical scavenger capacity. This subspecies is found in Tunisia and Algeria.

Origanum vulgare, subspecies hirtum, is the most

common Italian and Greek oregano. With strong and hardy growth, this subspecies is thought to be top tier for culinary purposes. It's grown not only in Greece, but in Cyprus, Turkey and the Balkans.

Origanum vulgare, subspecies viridulum, grows across a wide area, from Nepal to Corsica.

Origanum vulgare, subspecies virens, is also grown across many countries, including Spain, Portugal, Morocco, the Balearic Islands, the Canary Islands, Madeira and Azores.

Origanum vulgare, subspecies vulgare, is cultivated across Europe and Asia, and has even been naturalized in Venezuela and North America.

Chemical Components

Monoterpenes and monoterpenoids, which are high in antibacterial properties, make up most of oregano essential oil's chemical composition. Thymol and carvacrol make up the majority of the more than 60 chemical compounds found in oregano, as well as caryophyllene, germacrene-D, p-cymene, δ-terpineol, γ-terpinene, spathulenol, and β-fenchyl alcohol.

Volatile compounds are more highly concentrated at the end of the growing season and are also better fresh than dried, as the convection drying decreases and adversely affects the plant's compounds, sometimes by more than two thirds. It's important that these compounds remain intact, as they may help eliminate coughs, aid digestion, and fight against viruses, bacteria, fungi, and bodily parasites.

Main Properties of Oregano Essential Oil

Along with the antioxidant properties previously mentioned, oregano oil possesses antibacterial, antiviral, antifungal, anti-inflammatory, anti-allergenic, antiparasitic, emmenagogue, expectorant and digestive properties. Oregano is well equipped to fight off any pathogen or health issue in the body's path.

With a name like "oregano," which means "delight of the mountains" in Greek, it's no wonder that this mountain-grown herb was so popular amongst one of the greatest civilizations. The ancient Greeks were the first to identify oregano's antibacterial and disinfectant properties, using the herb to strengthen the body's natural defenses against wounds or skin infections, as well as to disinfect food. The oregano plant grew in high altitudes, which is where it acquired its name.

Oreganum vulgare, as mentioned, is composed of carvacrol, thymol, bisabolene, caryophyllene, pinene, linalyl acetate, cymene, linalool, terpinene, geranyl acetate and borneol. These components are what instill the enormously beneficial properties within oregano essential oil. We'll outline these properties below.

Antioxidant

Anything high in antioxidants – whether fruit, beans, or essential oils – is a powerful advocate for your body's health. Antioxidants both protect against free radicals and repair their damage. What are free radicals? Free radicals are destructive chemicals that invade your body, produced by substances both inside and out. Some free radicals (or oxidants) form through normal bodily reactions, like inflammation, metabolism and aerobic respiration. Other free radicals form outside the body, but enter it due to exposure. These include harmful pollutants, toxins, smoking, drinking alcohol, X-rays, and UV rays, to name a few. Although our bodies produce their own antioxidants, these often become damaged as we grow older; thus, introducing antioxidants into our bodies allow these nutrients and enzymes to assist in chemical reactions which destroy the oxidants or free radicals. Oregano essential oil, in particular, is composed of phenols, which is one of the strongest antioxidants, which detoxes the body of free radicals that lead to disease. Check out oregano's antioxidant activity in this study.

Antibacterial

Oregano's antibacterial properties make it a powerful protectant against diseases produced by bacteria, such as skin issues and infections, like urinary tract or colon infections. It can even combat cholera, typhoid and food poisoning. What's great is that, unlike some prescription drugs, oregano has no ill effects on bodily health or on the healthy natural flora that exists within the stomach and intestines. You can find further information about oregano's antibacterial properties here and here.

Antiviral

The antiviral protection that oregano essential oil grants will essentially empower the immune system, building up a tougher wall of security that most colds, measles or mumps are unlikely to scale. By boosting white blood cell count and function, this immune stimulant will ensure that your body is better prepared to protect against deadly viral infections.

Antifungal

While bacteria and viruses are plenty evil, fungi commonly lead to the most deadly infections, whether external or internal. Your ears, throat and nose are the most likely to become infected by fungi, the infections of which can be both excruciating and unsightly. If left untreated, fungal infections can kill, as they may spread to the brain. Oregano essential oil protects against these infections and more and is particularly effective against skin fungal infections. Read two studies examining oregano's antifungal properties here and here.

Anti-inflammatory

External or internal inflammation can be reduced

through the use of oregano. For instance, if you or your patient has swollen fingers from arthritis or a swollen knee from a sport's injury, topical application of oregano essential oil will decrease irritation or redness, while also soothing the pain that accompanies inflammation. You can take an oral capsule to provide a similar effect, though the pain may not be soothed as efficiently, as the oil must travel throughout the entire body. Follow this link to read a study on oregano's anti-inflammatory properties.

Anti-allergenic

Combining both the anti-inflammatory and sedative properties culminates in an anti-allergenic effect against hyperactive allergies or reactions to external catalysts. As a sedative, oregano calms the reaction and, as an anti-inflammatory, the allergy's severity is relieved and reduced. In the case of throat swelling, anaphylactic shock or other severe allergic reactions, this anti-allergenic effect is, quite literally, a life-saver.

Antiparasitic

Parasites include such mites as fleas, bedbugs, tapeworms, mosquitoes, and lice – pretty much any irritating insect, internal or external, which feeds off the body in one way or another. The human body is a tasty meal to parasites, which can sometimes lead to the transmission of communicable diseases through their feasting off various meals. Oregano is the answer. Its antiparasitic properties will combat mosquitoes, fleas, bedbugs and lice when applied topically, and intestinal worms when taken orally, which is why oregano is commonly used in insect repellents.

Emmenagogue

No need to look this one up. An emmenagogue is a menstrual stimulant for those with irregular menses. Oregano regulates hormones, which means that this emmenagogue can also delay and/or reduce the symptoms of menopause, which include hormonal and mood imbalance.

Expectorant

Throat or respiratory infections can be relieved through the use of oregano essential oil. Acting as an expectorant, oregano breaks up and helps destroy the phlegm and mucus buildup that accompanies sinuses or respiratory infections. Inflamed throat and lungs – and, thus, coughing – can also be relieved by the use of this oil.

Digestive

By boosting the production of absorptive enzymes, the digestibility of nutrients, and the secretion of digestive juices, oregano essential oil aids the digestive tract significantly, which can make a significant impact on your overall health by increasing those nutrients you absorb from food.

Common Medicinal Uses

Protecting Against Destructive Organisms

Oregano oil is purifying. Whether it comes to the toxins we take into our bodies on a daily basis or the accidental consumption of undercooked meat or impure water, oregano has shown the ability to detox the body of these destructive pathogens.

A 6-week study examined the correlation between the oral consumption of oregano oil and the elimination of bodily parasites. After six weeks, the parasites were entirely destroyed in those who daily took 600 mg of oregano essential oil. Oregano has been shown effective in fighting both inner parasites and external parasites – everything from tapeworms to lice, fleas and bedbugs.

Fighting the Common Cold

For those of us who are susceptible to seasonal cold and flu viruses (so...everyone), providing your immune system with a reliable mechanism of defense can mean the difference between illness and health. Oregano oil does just that – it protects your immune system and provides strong support when you need it most. You can take a precautionary measure by applying oregano orally with 3-6 drops in a capsule each day or, whenever you start falling ill, fill a capsule with 3-6 drops of the stuff daily before each meal, and you should see results within 5-10 days.

Providing Essential Nutrients

As with many essential oils, oregano is a strong source of the vitamins and minerals that are crucial to good health. These include vitamins C and E, as well as the minerals, zinc, iron, potassium copper, niacin, calcium, manganese and magnesium. The average human body is considerably deficient in these vitamins and minerals so, simply by administering oregano regularly, one can provide oneself with a boost of these essential nutrients.

Fighting Off Infection

A study from the Georgetown University Medical Center's Department of Physiology & Biophysics stated, "New, safe agents are needed to … overcome harmful organism infections. Based on our previous experience and that of others, we postulated that herbal essential oils, such as those of origanum (oregano oil)…offer such possibilities."

Many studies have concluded the same – oregano oil is a powerful antidote to infection. Used against staff infections, vaginal infections, aspergillus mold, candida albicans, and many other infectious strains, oregano has even been shown by the U.S. Department of Agriculture to combat E.coli and Salmonella.

Combating Fungal & Bacterial Infections

Skin fungal infections, such as athlete's foot, psoriasis,

and eczema, as well as bacterial infections, like giardiasis and e.coli, can all be targeted with oregano oil, due to the oil's impressive antifungal and antibacterial properties.

Relieving Aches & Pains

Oregano is also capable of addressing conditions that cause acute pain, such as backaches, carpal tunnel or arthritis. As a pain reliever, the oil can be topically applied to the affected area in a 50-50 mixture of oregano and a carrier oil (olive oil, for instance). This application should effectively relieve pain in everything from mild muscle stiffness to serious sport's injuries.

Aiding in Digestion

A healthy digestive tract means a healthy body, so maintaining good digestion can make a load of difference in how you feel, overall. Your digestive tract is between 25 and 30 feet long. If the length of it is not working properly, then there's a chance that food might get caught up and begin to rot within your body. Oregano effectively stops this buildup by inducing bile flow throughout the digestive organs, which will benefit your overall health.

Relieving Allergies

Bypass those allergy drugs with their laundry lists of side effects and, instead, seek out the therapeutic relief of oregano, which has been tested against allergic reactions with positive results, including a sedative effect and a soothing sense of relief to those with hyper-sensitive allergies.

Aiding Menstruation & Menopause

Women can particularly benefit from administering oregano if they commonly experience painful or irregular periods or unpleasant menopausal effects. Applying oregano can help young women become regular, relieve painful menstrual cramps, and combat unpleasant attributes of menopause, by better maintaining hormonal balance.

Combating the Effects of Aging

No need for those spliced-together anti-aging pills; oregano has been shown to help decelerate the process of aging, by fighting the deterioration of cells with its high number of antioxidants. Muscle degeneration, eye disease, and nervous disorders can all be protected against and targeted with the help of oregano oil.

Losing Weight

Those who need an extra boost to lose unwanted body fat can pop an oregano capsule, which has been shown to burn fat. This capability is due to oregano's high percentage of carvacrol, which both decreases irritation in white adipose tissue and also regulates genes. In mice, carvacrol also had the effect of lowering triglycerides and cholesterol levels.

Safety Precautions & Common Applications

Safety

Some adverse effects may evolve when using pure essential oils. Some essential oils should not be used when pregnant, for example, as they may cause miscarriage. Allergic reactions, too, may occur, especially when applied topically. Always administer an allergy test before committing fully to topical application. When used with other medications, essential oils may react negatively. If you are on any current prescription medications or have a chronic illness, such as high blood pressure, epilepsy or liver disease, then researching the effects of essential oils against your own personal medical history will eliminate any potentially problematic issues.

Oregano essential oil is a "hot" oil, which means it should be diluted no matter which application. Dilute in a 1:3 ratio (1 drop of oregano to 3 drops carrier oil), and further dilute if you have sensitive skin, as oregano may cause irritation. Below are further safety precautions:

- Do not use this oil for children under 6.

- Do not put in eyes, ears or nose.

- You may experience mild stomach upset when taking oregano.

- If you are allergic to plants in the Lamiaceae family – basil, lavender, hyssop, mint, marjoram, and sage – do not take oregano, as it may cause you to have a reaction.

- If pregnant or breast-feeding, consult with your doctor before usage. Large amounts may cause miscarriage.

- Do not take oregano if you have a bleeding disorder, as it may increase the risk.

- Do not take oregano if you have diabetes, as it may reduce blood sugar levels.

- Do not take oregano preceding a surgery, as it may increase bleeding. Stop using at least two weeks prior to surgery.

Blends

Oftentimes, essential oils are manufactured as blends of several pure oils. For instance, the Protective Essential Oil Blend is a mix of oregano, cinnamon, clove, rosemary, and eucalyptus. This blend can be used to boost the immune system to help support the body's defenses against colds, viruses and flus. The downside to blends is that the more oils added to the mix, the higher the probability your patient may react negatively to the blend if he/she is prone to allergies. There is also the possibility of phototoxicity when working with blends.

Regardless of these possible effects, essential oils are a viable option for support the body's defenses against a number of conditions. Those looking to enhance the maintenance of their own personal health, or that of their family's, should become educated on the uses of essential oils, their natural remedies and the methods of application. Only then can you begin building your kit of essential oils for survival.

Chapter 2:
Recipes for Oregano Essential Oil

In this chapter, we'll offer various recipes for oregano essential oil, both for pure oregano supportive remedies and for blends which incorporate the oil. For pure supportive remedies, we've provided the appropriate application and dosage to target specific ailments, from athlete's foot to whooping cough. When it comes to blends, herbalists and aromatherapists often combine oregano essential oil with bergamot, cypress, tea tree, lavender, chamomile, rosemary, eucalyptus, and cedar wood. We'll offer some fantastic supportive blending options in the second half of this chapter.

Pure Supportive Remedies

Athlete's Foot

Dilute oregano essential oil with a carrier oil and massage your feet. You can also add two drops of oregano to a foot bath or soak a pair of socks in warm water with two drops of oregano and wear them for a half hour. Place one drop in shoes to rid of contact fungus and for extended support.

Body Warmth

Oregano can serve to warm the body. Simply dilute oregano essential oil with a carrier oil and massage into hands, feet and around the neck.

Calluses

To rid of calluses, dilute oregano essential oil with a carrier oil and massage into the affected area daily.

Candida

Eliminate candida by diluting oregano essential oil with a carrier oil and massaging over affected area. You can also take oregano orally, through use in a capsule or as a food additive.

Canker Sores

Dilute oregano essential oil with a carrier oil and dab onto the sore 1-3 times daily, until the sore disappears.

Carpal Tunnel Syndrome

To relieve carpal tunnel syndrome, dilute oregano essential oil with a carrier oil and, in an upward movement (toward the heart), massage into the wrists, hands, forearms, upper arms, and shoulders.

Fungal Infections

Depending on the type of fungal infection, combat it through internal, topical, or aromatic application, according to its location. For instance, if you have athlete's foot, topical application may be the easiest and most direct solution. If you have an internal fungal infection, oral application would be more appropriate.

Immune System (Stimulant)

To boost the immune system, a variety of applications work well. You might try adding a drop of oregano essential oil to your meals. You can also apply topically by diluting it with carrier oil and massaging the combo into your feet. A third option is to place a few drops in your bathwater. And, lastly, you can use as an inhalant through steaming one drop in a pan of boiling water; remove the water from the stove and breathe in.

Inflammation

To relieve inflammation, dilute oregano essential oil with a carrier oil and massage toward the affected area toward the heart.

Intestinal Parasites

Intestinal parasites can be eliminated through internal or external use of oregano essential oil. Either take orally through capsules, add a drop of oregano to each meal, or dilute oregano essential oil with a carrier oil and massage into the abdomen in a clockwise rotation, as well as into the soles of the feet.

MRSA is an infection that results from a strain of staph bacteria which is now resistant to common antibiotics. You can support the body's natural defenses against it with oregano essential oil by diluting with a carrier oil and massaging over the chest and into the soles of the feet. This will simultaneously fight off the infection and stimulate immune response.

Muscle Aches

To relieve sore muscles, dilute oregano essential oil with a carrier oil and massage the solution into the affected area, toward the heart.

Nasal Polyp

Nasal polyps can be combated topically or through a

steam. If applying topically to the feet's reflex points, dilute oregano essential oil with a carrier oil. If you'd prefer the steam method, steam two drops of oregano essential oil in a pan of water, remove the steaming pan from the stove, pour into a bowl, place a towel over your head and inhale. If you don't feel it's done its job the first time, you can reheat that same water and use it once more without adding more oil.

Parasites

To combat parasites, take orally in either capsules, add a drop to your meals, or apply externally, diluting the oregano essential oil with a carrier oil and massaging into the soles of the feet or over the affected area.

Plague

Protect against and help relieve symptoms of the plague by diluting oregano essential oil with a carrier oil and massaging into the soles of the feet or by diffusing throughout the home.

Pneumonia

Help support the body's natural defenses against pneumonia by diluting oregano essential oil with a carrier oil and massaging into the soles of the feet or diffusing throughout the house. If you'd prefer the steam method, steam two drops of oregano essential oil in a pan of water, remove the steaming pan from the stove, pour into a bowl, place a towel over your head and inhale.

Ringworm

Ringworm can be targeted topically by diluting oregano essential oil with a carrier oil and massaging over the affected area three times a day. Once the ringworm is eliminated, continue the application for 3-5 days following recovery.

Staph Infection

Support the body's natural defenses against staph infections by diluting oregano essential oil with a carrier oil and massaging into the soles of the feet. This will cause your body to absorb the oil faster. You can also take capsules orally or add a drop into each meal.

Vaginal Candida

Vaginal candida can be targeted internally or externally. You may either take an oral capsule, add a drop to each meal, or apply internally with a vaginal syringe. Topically, you can dilute oregano essential oil with a carrier oil and massage into the soles of the feet.

Viral Infections

Strengthen the body's immunity against viral infections by diluting oregano essential oil with a carrier oil and massaging into the reflex points of the feet. Or, you can also place a few drops in your bathwater or apply a hot compress.

Warts

To eliminate warts, dilute oregano essential oil with a carrier oil and apply directly to the wart. Continue this application until the wart is removed.

Whooping Cough

Combat whooping cough by diluting oregano essential oil with a carrier oil and massaging into the soles of the feet and across the chest. You can also diffuse the oil throughout the home.

Blends

Protective Immune Support Blend (Antibiotic-Like)

Ingredients

- 2 drops Oregano Essential Oil

- 2 drops Wild Orange Peel Essential Oil

- 2 drops Black Pepper Seed Essential Oil

- 2 drops Cinnamon Bark Essential Oil

- 2 drops Clove Bud Essential Oil

- 2 drops Eucalyptus Leaf Essential Oil

- 2 drops Rosemary Essential Oil

- 2 drops Melissa Leaf Essential Oil* (Optional)

- 2 drops Lemon Essential Oil* (Optional)

Directions

For a general antibiotic, place all ingredients into a "00" capsule, and ingest 1 capsule three times a day.

Bladder Infection Support

Ingredients

- 6 drops Oregano Essential Oil

- 6 drops Protective Essential Oil Blend

- 2 drops Frankincense Essential Oil

Directions

To help relieve bladder infections, place all ingredients into a "00" capsule, and ingest 1 capsule three times a day. Additionally, you may ingest alongside ½ cup natural unsweetened cranberry juice to boost effectiveness.

Candida Cleanse

Ingredients

- 3 drops Oregano Essential Oil

- 5 drops Melaleuca Essential Oil

- 5 drops Lemon Essential Oil

Directions

To combat candida, place all ingredients into a "00" capsule, and ingest 1 capsule twice a day for a two-week period. Leave off the application for two weeks, and then repeat.

Colds I

Ingredients

- 3 drops Frankincense Essential Oil

- 5 drops Protective Essential Oil Blend

- 8 drops Oregano Essential Oil

Directions

To stave off colds or relieve cold symptoms, place all ingredients into a "00" capsule, and ingest 1 capsule twice a day.

Colds II

Ingredients

- 5 drops Oregano Essential Oil
- 5 drops Thyme Essential Oil
- 8 drops Clove Essential Oil

Directions

To stave off colds or relieve cold symptoms, place all ingredients into a "00" capsule, and ingest 1 capsule twice a day.

Cracked Heels

Ingredients

- ¼ cup Coconut Oil

- ¼ cup Shea Butter

- ¼ cup Magnesium Flakes (combined with 2 Tbsp boiling water)

- 3 Tbsp Beeswax

- 10 drops Peppermint Essential Oil

- 10 drops Oregano Essential Oil

Instructions

In a small bowl, combine 2 tablespoons boiling water with magnesium flakes to dissolve. The combination will be thick. Set aside. Place a mason jar in a small pan filled with 1 inch of water. Over medium heat, place beeswax, coconut oil, and shea butter in the mason jar and mix until melted and well combined. Remove the jar and let sit until liquid reaches room temperature. Pour contents into a blender and blend on medium speed. Slowly add the magnesium combo, one drop at a time, until well combined. Mix in the peppermint and oregano essential oils, whipping until blended. Place mixture in the refrigerator for 15 minutes then blend again, until mixture is a butter-like consistency. To apply, massage a thick coat into your cracked heels and wear socks until well absorbed. Store remainder in the fridge.

Dysentery

Ingredients

- 5 drops Digestive Support Essential Oil Blend (Ginger, Peppermint, Tarragon, Fennel, Caraway, Coriander, Anise)

- 5 drops Oregano Essential Oil

Directions

To combat dysentery, place all ingredients into a "00" capsule, and ingest 1 capsule three times a day for 2-4 weeks.

Flu Season Immune Support

Ingredients

- 2 drops Clove Essential Oil

- 2 drops Lemon Essential Oil

- 3 drops Frankincense Essential Oil

- 8 drops Oregano Essential Oil

Directions

To support the body's natural defenses against the flu, place all ingredients into a "00" capsule, and ingest 1 capsule twice a day.

Flu Season Immune Support II

Ingredients

- 2 drops Frankincense Essential Oil

- 6 drops Oregano Essential Oil

- 2 drops Protective Essential Oil Blend

Directions

To support the body's natural defenses against the flu, place all ingredients into a "00" capsule, and ingest 1 capsule every four hours for the first three day. If symptoms do not disappear, continue ingesting 1 capsule every eight hours for 4-6 days.

Immune Booster

Ingredients

- 10 drops Oregano Essential Oil

- 10 drops Protective Essential Oil Blend

- 20 drops Extra Virgin Olive Oil

Directions

To boost the immune system, place all ingredients into a roll-on bottle and apply to the soles of the feet.

Liver Cleanse Support

Ingredients

- 4 drops Rosemary Essential Oil

- 4 drops Lemongrass Essential Oil

- 4 drops Grapefruit Essential Oil

Directions

To cleanse the liver, place all ingredients into a "00" capsule, and ingest 1 capsule a day.

Parasitic Infections

Ingredients

- 1 drop Oregano Essential Oil

- 1 drop Melaleuca Essential Oil

- 1 drop Lemon Essential Oil

- 3 drops Protective Essential Oil Blend

Directions

To fight off parasitic infections, place all ingredients into a "00" capsule, and ingest 1 capsule twice a day for 10-14 days.

Sinuses

Ingredients

- 3 drops Rosemary Essential Oil

- 3 drops Oregano Essential Oil

- 3 drops Protective Essential Oil Blend

- 2 drops Myrrh Essential Oil

- 2 drops Frankincense Essential Oil

Directions

To clear sinuses, place all ingredients into a "00" capsule, and ingest 1 capsule 1-3 times a day or as needed. Continue taking for 2 days after symptoms subside.

Staph Infection or MRSA

Ingredients

- 1 drop Frankincense Essential Oil

- 4 drops Melaleuca Essential Oil

- 4 drops Oregano Essential Oil

Directions

To combat staph infection or MRSA, place all ingredients into a "00" capsule, and ingest 1 capsule 2-3 times a day.

Stomach Ulcer Support

Ingredients

- 2 drops Oregano Essential Oil

- 2-3 drops Peppermint Essential Oil

- 10 drops Lemongrass Essential Oil

Directions

To eliminate a stomach ulcer, place all ingredients into a "00" capsule, and ingest 1 capsule a day.

Urinary Tract Infection

Ingredients

- 6 drops Oregano Essential Oil

- 6 drops Protective Essential Oil Blend

- 2 drops Frankincense Essential Oil

Directions

To help support the body's natural defenses against bladder infection, place all ingredients into a "00" capsule, and ingest 1 capsule three times a day. Additionally, you may ingest alongside ½ cup natural unsweetened cranberry juice to boost the application's effectiveness.

Chapter 3:
Oregano Essential Oil Studies

Many studies have been done on essential oils to uncover and prove their therapeutic qualities. In the case of the great number of oregano studies, many of the properties attributed to the essential oil (noted in this book and elsewhere) are quite often validated through the scientific research of accredited universities and published by accredited scientific journals. In this chapter, we'll discuss a small portion of this research. It's important to note that research on essential oils is constant and evolving. Keep up with any recent studies, as they may turn up even further valuable uses of these miracle oils.

Study 1 – Antifungal Properties

In this study published by the Brazilian Journal of Microbiology, the antifungal effects of the oil were examined, with the following results: "The aim of this study was to evaluate the in vitro activity of the essential oil extracted from Origanum vulgare against sixteen Candida species isolates. Standard strains tested comprised C. albicans (ATCC strains 44858, 4053, 18804 and 3691), C. parapsilosis (ATCC 22019), C. krusei (ATCC 34135), C. lusitaniae (ATCC 34449) and C. dubliniensis (ATCC MY646)...All isolates tested in vitro were sensitive to O. vulgare essential oil...The antifungal activity of O. vulgare essential oil against Candida spp. observed in vitro suggests its administration may represent an alternative treatment for candidiasis."

Candidiasis, in layman's terms, is yeast infection. Thus, the study's results confirm the claims of successful application of oregano essential oil against vaginal candida and other candida infections.

Reference
http://www.ncbi.nlm.nih.gov/pubmed/24031471]

http://www.ncbi.nlm.nih.gov/pmc/articles/PMC3768597/pdf/bjm-41-116.pdf]

Study 2 – Antimicrobial Activity

In this study published by The Scientific World Journal, the antimicrobial effects of oregano essential oil were examined, with the following results: "The effect of solvent polarity (methanol and pentane) on the chemical composition of hydrodistilled essential oils (EO's) of Lippia graveolens H.B.K. (MXO) and Origanum vulgare L. (EUO) was studied by GC-MS...The antimicrobial activity of free and microencapsulated EO's was evaluated. They were tested against Salmonella sp., Brochothrix thermosphacta, Pseudomonas fragi, Lactobacillus plantarum, and Micrococcus luteus...Microencapsulation retains most antimicrobial activity and improves stability of EO's from oregano."

To better explain this study, it's imperative to know that all of the above mentioned bacteria tested are common food spoilage bacterium present in everything from dairy to meat to vegetables. The research shows that oregano essential oil's antimicrobial activity was retained and its stability improved after microencapsulation. Microencapsulation is a process in which small particles (or, in this case, essential oils) are provided a coating so that they may form a capsule, assumably to ingest orally. This is done to designate proper dosing and prevent the breakdown of pharmaceuticals.

Reference
http://www.ncbi.nlm.nih.gov/pubmed/25177730]

Study 3 – Antibacterial Properties

In this study published by Molecules journal, the antibacterial effects of oregano essential oil were examined, with the following results: "This research was aimed at investigating the essential oil production, chemical composition and biological activity of a crop of pink flowered oregano (Origanum vulgare L. subsp. vulgare L.) under different spatial distribution of the plants (single and binate rows)...The essential oils showed antimicrobial action, mainly against Gram-positive pathogens and particularly Bacillus cereus and B. subtilis."

Bacillus cereus is an endemic, Gram-positive bacterium that dwells in the soil, and certain strains can cause foodborne illness. It's sometimes called "fried rice syndrome," due to the fact that this bacteria is commonly contracted from fried rice that's been left out for hours on end (like at a buffet). In this study, oregano essential oil, yet again, is shown to combat various bacteria, including this one.

Reference
http://www.ncbi.nlm.nih.gov/pubmed/24304588]

http://www.mdpi.com/1420-3049/18/12/14948#tabs-5]

Study 4 – Anti-inflammatory Properties

In this study published by Mediators of Information, the anti-inflammatory effects of oregano essential oil were examined, with the following results: "We examined the anti-inflammatory effects of the combination of thyme and oregano essential oil dietary administered at three concentrations (0.4% thyme and 0.2% oregano oils; 0.2% thyme and 0.1% oregano oils; 0.1% thyme and 0.05% oregano oils) on mice with TNBS-induced colitis...Our results indicate that combined treatment with appropriate concentrations of thyme and oregano essential oils can reduce the production of proinflammatory cytokines, and thereby attenuate TNBS-induced colitis in mice."

Colitis is a chronic or acute digestive disease in which the colon is inflamed. This study confirms the use of oregano essential oil in combating colitis. Oregano is also an effective application for other digestive issues.

Reference
http://www.ncbi.nlm.nih.gov/pubmed/18288268]

http://www.ncbi.nlm.nih.gov/pmc/articles/PMC2233768/pdf/MI2007-23296.pdf]

Study 5 – Antimalarial & Anticancer

In this study published by Cytotechnology, the antimicrobial effects of oregano essential oil were examined, with the following results: "GC-FID and GC-MS analysis of essential oil from oregano leaves (Origanum compactum) resulted in the identification of 46 compounds, representing more than 98% of the total composition...The samples (essential oil and extracts) were subjected to a screening for antioxidant (DPPH and ABTS assays) and antimalarial activities and against human breast cancer cells. The essential oil showed a higher antioxidant activity with an IC50=2±0.1 mg/L. Among the extracts, the aqueous extract had the highest antioxidant activity with an IC50=4.8±0.2 mg/L (DPPH assay). Concerning antimalarial activity, Origanum compactum essential oil and ethyl acetate extract showed the best results with an IC50 of 34 and 33 mg/mL, respectively. In addition, ethyl acetate extract (30 mg/L) and ethanol extract (56 mg/L) showed activity against human breast cancer cells (MCF7). The oregano essential oil was considered to be nontoxic."

In summary, this study indicates that oregano essential oil ("compactum," not the more common "vulgare") is an effective antidote to malaria, the mosquito-borne infectious disease, and also against human breast cancer cells.

Reference
http://www.ncbi.nlm.nih.gov/pubmed/21535822]http://www.ncbi.nlm.nih.gov/pmc/articles/PMC3261448/pdf/10616_2011_Article_9389.pdf]

Study 6 – Antifungal Properties

In this study published by Frontiers in Microbiology, the antifungal effects of oregano essential oil were examined, with the following results: "Inhibitory effects of essential oils of Ageratum conyzoides (mentrasto) and Origanum vulgare (oregano) on the mycelial growth and aflatoxin B1 production by Aspergillus flavus have been studied previously in culture medium. The aim of this study was to evaluate aflatoxin B1 production by Aspergillus flavus in real food systems (corn and soybean) treated with Ageratum conyzoides (mentrasto) and Origanum vulgare (oregano) essential oils. Fungal growth and aflatoxin production were inhibited by essential oils, but the mentrasto oil was more effective in soybeans than that of oregano. The results indicate that both essential oils can become an alternative for the control of aflatoxins in corn and soybeans."

Aflatoxin B1 (AFB1) is a toxic and carcinogenic mycotoxin produced in food by the Aspergillus species. This study shows that oregano essential oil effectively destroys the fungal growth and has the potential to control the infestation of aflatoxins in soybeans and corn.

Reference
http://www.ncbi.nlm.nih.gov/pubmed/24926289]

http://www.ncbi.nlm.nih.gov/pmc/articles/PMC4044670/pdf/fmicb-05-00269.pdf]

Study 7 – Food Preservation

In this study published by the Journal of Applied Microbiology, the antimicrobial effects of oregano essential oil were examined, with the following results: "The minimum inhibitory concentration (MIC) of oregano essential oil (OEO) and two of its principle components, i.e. thymol and carvacrol, against Pseudomonas aeruginosa and Staphylococcus aureus was assessed by using an innovative technique. The mechanism of action of the above substances was also investigated...Mixing carvacrol and thymol at proper amounts may exert the total inhibition that is evident by oregano essential oil. Such inhibition is due to damage in membrane integrity, which further affects pH homeostasis and equilibrium of inorganic ions...The knowledge of extent and mode of inhibition of specific compounds, which are present in plant extracts, may contribute to the successful application of such natural preservatives in foods, since certain combinations of carvacrol-thymol provide as high inhibition as oregano essential oil with a smaller flavour impact."

This study shows the potential for oregano essential oil use as a natural food preservative. This means that oregano could increase a product's shelf-life, as well as improve the chances of safe consumption.

Reference
http://www.ncbi.nlm.nih.gov/pubmed/11556910]

http://onlinelibrary.wiley.com/doi/10.1046/j.1365-

Study 8 – Insecticidal

In this study published by the Journal of Animal Science, the insecticidal effects of oregano essential oil were examined, with the following results: "This study analysed the chemical constituents and bioactivity of essential oils that were isolated via hydrodistillation from Origanum vulgare L. (oregano) and Thymus vulgaris L. (thyme) against eggs, second instar and adults of Nezara viridula (L.)...Both oils produced repellency on nymphs and adults...These results showed that the essential oils from O. vulgare and T. vulgaris could be applicable to the management of N. viridula."

Nezara viridula are green plant-feeding stink bugs, prominent in the south of the United States, as well as in Australia and New Zealand. The effect of oregano essential oil on these pests has shown to be destructive, making oregano a powerful natural insecticide.

Reference
http://www.ncbi.nlm.nih.gov/pubmed/21394885]

http://www.journalofanimalscience.org/content/89/4/1079.full.pdf+html]

Chapter 4:
The Ins & Outs of Essential Oils

Where do essential oils come from?

Plants and plant species naturally produce essential oils for various reasons, one being to draw pollinator insects to them, another being to repel invading organisms (bacteria, animals). A number of chemical compounds compose each plant's essential oil, and the combination of these compounds is specific to each oil, which then instills in the oil its own unique properties. Essential oils can be harnessed from all sorts of plant components, including flowers, leaves, bark, fruit, roots, and resin. For instance, cinnamon oil is harnessed from bark, lemon oil from the peel, and lavender oil from lavender flowers. Certain plants can produce a few chemical variants of the same essential oil, which are acquired from different parts of the plant. Some of these parts produce a large amount of oil, while others produce just a smidgen. The oil's quality and potency depends upon a number of factors, including the subspecies of the plant, its soil conditions, the time of year and even the time of day you harvest it.

How are essential oils extracted?

Essential oils can be extracted from plants through various methods, including pressing, distillation, solvent and maceration. Let's take a brief look at each:

Pressing Method

Commonly used with citrus fruit, the pressing method extracts the oil through a technique which involves pushing the fruit peels through a press. Oily fruits and plants are best suited for this technique. Orange oil, for example, is extracted from orange skins through the pressing method.

Distillation Method

This technique harkens back to the days of old-timey moonshiners, as the same sort of method used to create strong liquor can be used to extract essential oils. Using a still, boiled water and plant materials will create steam which is then cooled by coils and condensed into a combination of water and oil. This combination doesn't mix, so the oil can then be extracted from it.

Solvent Method

Through a multi-step process, certain plant and flower oils can be extracted using alcohol and other solvents, which extort the essential oil from the plant materials.

Maceration Method

When a "carrier" or fixed oil or lard is mixed with the plant material and set out in the sun, over a period of time, the carrier oil is infused with the plant's essence. Heat sources, other than the sun, are often used to speed the process. Throughout the process, more plant material is added to produce a more potent oil.

How do you use essential oils?

Although some studies about the effectiveness of essential oils are conducted by small companies or even individuals, a number of them are conducted by the food and cosmetic industries. In general, the pharmaceutical industry shows next to no interest in herbal medicine, primarily because there are few options to patent such products. Being as such, the product's lack of profitability results in a lack of research funding. Regardless, the historical uses of essential oils tell us what we need to know: these oils have been effectively administered for centuries. The therapeutic qualifications of essential oils can be plotted in the survival of the human race across cultures and generations.

Another reason that studies on essential oils have not resulted in much conclusive evidence as to their overall effectiveness is because definitive results are sometimes difficult to prove, as the quality of each batch of oil can vary for a number of reasons. One is that essential oils are impossible to standardize. As mentioned above, even the slightest variance in soil conditions and the time of harvesting – as well as innumerable other factors – will produce a different product quality and potency. In addition, essential oils are often obtained from various species of the same plant; Eucalyptus radiata and Eucalyptus globulus can both be used in the making of therapeutic-grade eucalyptus oil and, as a result, they may have slightly different properties and degrees of strength or effectiveness.

Just as there are a number of methods by which to extract essential oils, there are a number of methods to administer them therapeutically. The variety of chemical compounds in each essential oil means that their benefits and applications also vary across the board. Below are a few of these methods.

Topical Administration

Direct application of many essential oils works like a sponge, as skin sops up chemicals and other things (like sunlight, for instance). Topical application is best when you want to clear up an ailment on the skin's surface or in the underlying muscle tissue. When applying topically, you may either massage the oil into the skin or simply dab on the skin for therapeutic results. You might combine the essential oil with a carrier oil for topical use in order to dilute its potency. This is safer, as the oil is so concentrated. You may support your body's defenses against rash or muscle pain in this manner, but you should always test your patient for allergies before applying. Adverse effects are produced by natural chemicals as much as synthetic ones; poison ivy, for example.

To test for allergens, place a drop or two on your patient's inner forearm. If a rash develops within 12 to 24 hours, then the patient is allergic. In addition, phototoxicity – sun exposure resulting in an exacerbated burn – may be an issue when citrus oils are applied topically. So one must proceed with caution when applying essential oils using this method.

Inhalation Therapy

Commonly known as "aromatherapy", this essential oil application is effective for inner ailments, like sore throat or cold. In a steaming bowl of distilled or sterilized water, add a few drops of essential oil and, with a towel over your head, bend over the bowl and inhale. The towel captures the vapors, making the technique even more effective. Essential oils can also be placed in a diffuser or potpourri throughout a room to produce somewhat diluted therapeutic effects.

Ingestion

When using this method, proceed with caution. Direct ingestion of essential oils must be monitored and applied in small doses that are diluted in a tablespoon or more of any carrier oil – olive oil, for example. If you are unsure of dosage amounts, make a tea with the relevant herb instead. Although the effects of this diluted use may be weaker, this application is a better alternative than an overdose of essential oils.

What are the general benefits of using essential oils?

Replacement for Prescription Drugs

One practical benefit for using essential oils is, of course, their substitutive nature; they can replace Rx drugs, which is the ultimate reason to educate yourself on their administration and to begin stockpiling your essential oil supply. One of the potential threats of economic or social collapse is the lack of resources, and primarily the inability to procure prescription drugs. Being as such, finding suitable supplements should be a priority when preparing for the worst.

Their portability is also a major bonus when it comes to survival prepping. The fact that these ultra-concentrated oils take up little-to-no space makes toting them to your shelter all the simpler should the need arise. And, because essential oils are highly concentrated, the application used in most methods of administration requires only a drop or two of oil, which means that tiny bottle will be long-lasting.

Cost Effective Supplement

Though money may be the last thing on your mind when it comes to prepping for a survival situation (money may even be obsolete in the event of social collapse), it is worth noting that the expense of essential oils pales in comparison to prescription drugs. Essential oils are a cost effective supplement to prescription medicine.

No Expiration Date

Another benefit of essential oils is that they do not expire, neither do they have "proper storage" requirements. A number of medicines and medicinal products must be replaced every couple years, so this sets essential oils ahead of the pack when it comes to shelf life.

Versatility

Essential oils also offer great versatility. Apart from providing therapeutic benefits, essential oils can be repurposed for household and hygienic applications. For instance, if you're looking for something that might serve your dental hygiene needs in a time of crisis, the protective oil blend is your go-to essential oil. If you want to maintain your skin's tone and condition, frankincense and lavender will do the trick; the latter also serves as sunscreen, so you can inhibit sun damage as well.

When it comes to the house or shelter, you can use essential oils to deodorize, which will come in handy in a disaster scenario where things might start to smell fishy due to lack of proper utilities and care. For example, after the 2011 tsunami and the subsequent nuclear reactor meltdown in Japan, a nurse named Risa Nakahira used essential oils to deodorize and sanitize putrid public bathrooms in overpopulated evacuation facilities. As relief workers searched for survivors, often wading through debris and decay, Nakahira also deodorized their boots and masks using essential oils. The possibilities of these natural oils are endless.

They are also versatile when it comes to the range of patients they're capable of supporting. The wellness of everyone from your great grandfather to your infant baby can be fortified with the aid of essential oils in the appropriate dosage. They even come in handy when supporting the wellness of livestock or pets. From teething infants to dementia in the elderly, from teenagers with acne to dogs with urinary tract infections, essential oils can serve any patient with nearly any ailment.

Conclusion

Now that you know all about what oregano essential oil can do for you – where it originates, how it's extracted, its benefits and properties, and the different methods of administration – you can use it confidently to support the body's defenses against health issues and start to assemble a kit of essential oils for survival.

The various benefits of essential oils and their properties are countless. To build your own kit, first focus on acquiring the essential oils which may bear more relevance to your health issues or the potential health threats within your environment. When it comes to skin health, for instance, myrrh essential oil will be one of your more crucial oils, due to its antibacterial, anti-inflammatory, antifungal, and astringent properties.

Used as a supplement or as your go-to for immune system support, blood circulation, or gum and hair health, the application of myrrh essential oil in medicine has survived for centuries and will survive centuries more. When it comes down to it, you don't need to rely on pharmaceuticals; essential oils, herbs, and plenty of other natural ingredients can be used to help support any number of health issues, whether ailment or injury.

Essential oils are essential to your survival in the case of viral outbreak, social collapse or natural disaster because, when the SHTF, your access to pharmaceuticals will likely either be limited or eliminated altogether. Alternatives to our modern-day standard will equate survival when no other option exists. And when it comes to a life-or-death situation, you can't let your health decline, no matter the state of the world.

ALL RIGHTS RESERVED. No part of this publication may be reproduced or transmitted in any form whatsoever, electronic, or mechanical, including photocopying, recording, or by any informational storage or retrieval system without express written, dated and signed permission from the author.

DISCLAIMER AND/OR LEGAL NOTICES: Every effort has been made to accurately represent this book and it's potential. Results vary with every individual, and your results may or may not be different from those depicted. No promises, guarantees or warranties, whether stated or implied, have been made that you will produce any specific result from this book. Your efforts are individual and unique, and may vary from those shown. Your success depends on your efforts, background and motivation.

The material in this publication is provided for educational and informational purposes only and is not intended as medical advice. The information contained in this book should not be used to diagnose or treat any illness, metabolic disorder, disease or health problem. Always consult your physician or healthcare provider before beginning any nutrition or exercise program. Use of the programs, advice, and information contained in this book is at the sole choice and risk of the reader.

www.ingramcontent.com/pod-product-compliance
Lightning Source LLC
Chambersburg PA
CBHW062109280526
45788CB00003B/1410